THE ULTIMATE FIRST-TIME MOM'S PREGNANCY COOKBOOK

Nutrition Guide Recipes for Healthy Pregnancy

Adam C.

DEDICATION

This book is dedicated to all my Readers

CONTENTS

Introduction

Welcome to the Journey of Your Pregnancy

Congratulations on taking on one of the most amazing journeys of your life: parenting! Your pregnancy journey is full of expectation, joy, and maybe even a few fears if you're a first-time mother. The decisions you make for your health and wellbeing during this unique period affect not only you but also your developing child. To help you on this incredible journey, "The Ultimate First-Time Mom's Pregnancy Cookbook: Nutrition Guide Recipes for Healthy Pregnancy" is here.

The Importance of Nutrition during Pregnancy

Because pregnancy brings about such profound physical and psychological changes, it is more important than ever to maintain a healthy diet. Foods are very important for a healthy pregnancy, for the development of your unborn child, and for your general health. You may lessen discomfort, lower the chance of complications, and build a solid foundation for your baby's future by providing them with the correct nutrients.

We'll go into the importance of nutrition throughout pregnancy and how it can benefit both you and your unborn child in this eBook. We'll go over the most important nutrients for a healthy pregnancy and the value of a balanced diet so you can grasp the fundamental ideas behind our recipe development.

How to Use This Cookbook

On this amazing journey, "The Ultimate First-Time Mom's Pregnancy Cookbook" is your reliable friend. The main reason we created this eBook is to make sure you have access to a variety of tasty, nutritious, and simple-to-follow recipes while you're pregnant.

Here's how to make the most of this cookbook

- Discover the critical nutrients required throughout pregnancy by reading through our extensive nutrition guide.
- Explore a wide range of dishes that are appropriate for a pregnant woman, all carefully crafted to meet her specific dietary needs and preferences.

- Discover useful advice and ideas to make meal preparation and planning simple, especially on days when you might not feel your best.
- Savor a range of flavors to make sure your meals are not only filling and healthy but also pleasurable.

Our goal in writing this eBook is to provide you with the information and resources you need to make wise eating decisions while enjoying the delectable treats that will add even more special moments to your pregnancy. We hope your pregnancy is happy and healthy, and we are excited to be a part of your amazing journey.

Chapter 1: Building a Healthy Foundation

Your body is preparing for the amazing journey of pregnancy long before you see those two pink lines on the pregnancy test. A healthy and bright pregnancy is mostly determined by your nutrition and overall health during the first trimester and the months leading up to conception. This chapter will cover how to create a strong base for your pregnancy, starting with preconception nutrition and moving on to first trimester essentials.

1.1 Nutrition for Preconception

The path to parenting starts long before you become pregnant. It all begins with your preconception nutrition and lifestyle for a healthy pregnancy. If you intend to get pregnant, there are a few important things to think about:

1. Folate and Folic Acid: First, make sure your diet has adequate folate and folic acid. Folate is an essential B-vitamin that helps keep neural tube abnormalities in babies at bay. Foods such as citrus fruits, legumes, and leafy greens contain it. A doctor might suggest taking a folic acid supplement in specific situations.

2. Balanced Diet: Make an effort to eat a diet rich in a range of fruits, vegetables, whole grains, lean meats, dairy products, and dairy substitutes. This prepares you for consuming a balanced diet when you get pregnant.

3. Hydration: It's crucial to maintain adequate hydration at all times, but it's crucial when getting ready for pregnancy. Drinking enough water helps keep your body functioning optimally.

4. Minimize or Give Up Dangerous Habits: It's critical to give up smoking, drinking alcohol, and using recreational drugs well in advance of becoming pregnant because these behaviors can have a negative impact on the health of your unborn child.

5. Handle Chronic Conditions: Before getting pregnant, make sure your healthcare professional is helping you manage any chronic health issues you may have, such as high blood pressure or diabetes.

1.2 The Essentials of the First Trimester

When you get the happy news that you are expecting, your baby's first trimester is a time of rapid development. It's critical to continue eating a healthy diet during this period. Here are some crucial things to remember:

1. Morning Sickness: Morning sickness is a common side effect of pregnancy. Eat more often and in smaller portions to help manage it. Go for simple, digestible foods like soups, ginger tea, and crackers.

2. Folate Remains Critical: Given that neural tube development occurs early in the first trimester, it is important to keep eating foods high in folate.

3. Iron-Rich Foods: To maintain the increased blood volume during pregnancy, your body requires more iron. Include foods high in iron, such as spinach, lean meats, chicken, and beans, in your diet.

4. Protein for Growth: Your baby's development depends on protein. Add sources such as dairy, eggs, lean meats, and plant-based foods like lentils or tofu.

1.3 Preparing Your Body for Pregnancy

In addition to diet, the following actions should be taken in the first trimester and before conception to make sure your body is prepared for the voyage ahead:

1. Prenatal Supplements: For information on prenatal supplements, speak with your doctor. During the first trimester, these can assist guarantee that you're getting the vitamins and minerals you need.

2. Frequent Exercise: To keep your body strong and maintain a healthy weight, engage in moderate physical activity. Consult your healthcare physician about your fitness regimen to be sure it is appropriate for pregnant.

3. Stress management: Since pregnancy brings about both physical and emotional changes, engage in stress-reduction exercises like yoga or meditation.

4. Sleep: Make sleep a priority in order to maintain your general wellbeing. You can feel tired, so it's important to get enough rest.

Establishing a sound basis for your pregnancy is a wonderful present for your unborn child and yourself. You're laying the groundwork for a gorgeous and healthy trip ahead with the appropriate dietary and lifestyle decisions. We'll explore tasty and nourishing recipes in the upcoming chapters, which will add to the enjoyment of this voyage.

Chapter 2: Foods High in Nutrients for Pregnancy

Your growing baby and you are both greatly impacted by the dietary decisions you make during your pregnancy. We'll discuss the key nutrients required for pregnancy in this chapter, along with how to include them in your diet. We'll concentrate on folate, folic acid, iron, calcium, and the need of drinking plenty of water during this amazing journey.

2.1 Essential Nutrients for Mom and Baby

Your body needs a variety of vital nutrients as it sets out on the incredible path of supporting a new life. It is crucial that you and your child acquire these essential elements:

1. Folate and Folic Acid: Folate is an essential B-vitamin that helps shield your unborn child from neural tube abnormalities. Although natural sources of folate include citrus fruits, lentils, and leafy greens, many medical professionals advise taking a folic acid supplement when pregnant.

2. Iron: During pregnancy, your body need more iron since it is necessary for the blood to carry oxygen. To fulfill your iron needs, include lean meats, poultry, fortified cereals, and dark green vegetables in your diet.

3. Calcium: Your baby's growing teeth and bones depend on calcium. Good sources of calcium include dairy products, leafy greens, and fortified plant-based milk.

4. Protein: Your baby's growth is supported by protein. A diet rich in lean meats, poultry, fish, eggs, dairy products, legumes, and nuts guarantees a sufficient intake of protein.

5. Fiber: During pregnancy, constipation is a typical problem that fiber helps prevent. Good sources of fiber include fruits, vegetables, whole grains, and legumes.

2.2 Incorporating Folate and Folic Acid

Naturally occurring in food, folate is an essential nutrient for pregnant women. Leafy greens, citrus fruits, and beans abound. However, because it can be difficult to obtain the recommended quantity from diet alone, many pregnant women additionally require folic acid supplements. To make sure you're getting adequate folic acid and folate, try these methods:

1. Leafy Greens: Increase the amount of collard, kale, and spinach in your salads and dishes.

2. Citrus Fruits: Oranges, grapefruits, and lemons are examples of citrus fruits that can be enjoyed as a nutritious and revitalizing snack.

3. Legumes: Lentils and beans are great providers of folate. Add them to salads, stews, and soups.

4. Foods Fortified: Folic acid is added to a lot of breads, pastas, and breakfast cereals. Look for additional nutrients on labels.

2.3 Calcium, Iron, and Other Things

Two more important minerals that are crucial during pregnancy are iron and calcium. How to include them in your meals is as follows:

1. Iron-Rich Meals: Fish and poultry, which are lean meats, are excellent providers of iron. Lentils, beans, and tofu are examples of plant-based alternatives. To improve the absorption of iron, combine these with meals high in vitamin C, such as strawberries or bell peppers.

2. Dairy and Fortified Milk: Dairy products contain calcium, including milk, cheese, and yogurt. Choose fortified plant-based milk substitutes if you eat a plant-based diet.

3. Hydration and Pregnancy: It's important to drink enough of water during your pregnancy. Water is vital for your baby's development and is involved in almost all bodily processes. Try to have eight to ten glasses of water a day, or more if it's extremely hot outside or you're active.

Herbal teas and fresh fruit juices can be delightful alternatives to water. Steer clear of caffeine in excess as it can cause dehydration.

As you embark on this incredible journey, never forget that the meals you eat are essential for maintaining the health of both you and your unborn child. This eBook's recipes have been thoughtfully created to satisfy your palate and help you achieve your dietary goals. Watch for additional dishes that are safe to make during pregnancy in the upcoming chapters.

Chapter 3: Remedies for Morning Sickness

Morning sickness is a common companion throughout the early stages of pregnancy for many pregnant women. Mealtimes can be difficult when nausea and vomiting are present, but there are techniques and dishes that can help you manage this common pregnancy symptom. This chapter will address how to deal with morning sickness, include some recipes that may help with nausea, and stress the value of being hydrated.

3.1 Handling Morning Illness

There are different levels of morning sickness: mild queasiness to extreme nausea and vomiting. Even though it's commonly called "morning" sickness, it can happen at any time of day. Here are some coping mechanisms to assist you manage this typical pregnant symptom:

1. Regular, Small Meals: Eating more often and in smaller portions will help prevent your stomach from being overly empty, which can cause nausea. Between meals, munch on some toast, crackers, or fresh fruit.

2. Ginger: Ginger naturally possesses anti-nausea qualities. To assist ease nausea, try ginger tea, ginger candies, or foods that contain ginger.

3. Acupressure Bands: Acupressure wristbands, which apply pressure to a certain area on the wrist that is thought to help alleviate nausea, can provide comfort for certain women.

4. Avoid Triggers: Certain meals, images, or odors can make someone sick. Determine what personally triggers you, and try to stay away from them.

5. Stay Upright After Eating: Refrain from dozing off right away. Stomach acid can cause nausea, but being upright can help stop it from pouring back into the esophagus.

3.2 Recipes Suitable for Nausea

Selecting foods that are easy on the stomach is crucial when you're suffering from morning sickness. Here are some recipes to think about:

Smoothie with bananas and oatmeal:

Components:

- One mature banana
- Oats, half a cup rolled
- 1 cup of yogurt, plain
- One tablespoon of honey

Instructions: Purée all ingredients until well combined. This smoothie is simple to digest and gives you energy and nutrition without making you feel bloated.

Sweet potatoes mashed:

Components:

- Two sweet potatoes, medium
- Two tablespoons of margarine or butter
- A dash of cinnamon, if desired

Instructions: Sweet potatoes should be boiled until tender, and then mashed with butter and a dash of cinnamon. This is a mildly flavored, wholesome side dish that goes well with anything.

Tea with ginger and honey:

Ingredients:

- 1 inch of freshly peeled and sliced ginger
- One tablespoon of honey

Instructions: Boil slices of ginger in water, drain, and then stir in honey. This calming tea helps relieve nausea.

3.3 Continuing to Drink

Dehydration can result from nausea and vomiting, which is especially dangerous when pregnant. Health problems such as weariness and dizziness can be brought on by dehydration. Keeping hydrated:

- Drink water all day, even if you can only take a few little swallows at a time.
- Try drinking clear, hydrating beverages like watermelon juice, ginger ale, or coconut water.
- To stay hydrated, try ice pops, chips, or cubes with fruit flavors.

Never forget that if your morning sickness gets worse or you can't take any food or liquids down, you need to talk to your doctor.

They may offer advice and guarantee the health of both you and your child.

Even though morning sickness might be difficult, it's frequently a passing stage of pregnancy. These techniques and mild, nausea-inducing dishes will help you more effectively manage this part of your pregnancy. We'll continue to look at tasty and healthful dishes that will benefit the wellbeing of you and your infant in the upcoming chapters.

Chapter 4: Second Trimester Delights

Pregnancy's second trimester is frequently accompanied with a flurry of novel possibilities and experiences. Because they frequently feel more energized and their pregnancy symptoms, such morning sickness, tend to lessen, many women believe that this stage is more joyful. This chapter will discuss how to enjoy the most of your second trimester by trying new foods, exercising to maintain your fitness level even with a growing baby belly, and indulging in recipes that will give you more energy.

4.1 Investigating Novel Tastes

Your taste may become more daring than usual in the second trimester. Hormonal shifts can enhance your perception of taste and smell, which makes now an excellent moment to try out new flavors and culinary traditions. Here are some concepts to think about:

1. International Cuisine: Indulge your appetites with delectable foods from around the world, such as robust Italian pastas and fiery Thai curries.

2. Options for Vegetarians and Vegans: Try out several plant-based meals with a wide range of tastes and textures. This can be a fantastic chance for you to eat more fruits, veggies, and legumes.

3. Seasonal Ingredients: Cook with fresh, locally obtained ingredients to embrace the flavors of the moment. In addition to having a greater flavor, seasonal fruits and vegetables are frequently healthier.

4. Combinations of Sweet and Savory Flavors: Experiment with the wonderful contrast between sweet and savory flavors. Consider dressing up your salads with savory components like cheese or grilled chicken and fruits like mango or apple.

4.2 Baby Bum-Friendly Exercise Plans

Maintaining an active lifestyle during pregnancy can help you feel your best and get your body ready for giving birth. The following are some safe and gentle workouts for your growing baby bump:

1. Prenatal Yoga: Classes focused on prenatal yoga are created with expectant mothers in mind. These courses emphasize breathing exercises, relaxation, and flexibility all of which can be quite helpful before, during, and after childbirth.

2. Swimming: Swimming is a full-body, low-impact exercise that relieves the extra weight of pregnancy and is easy on the joints.

3. Walking: Getting regular exercise can be achieved with just a few easy steps. It's simple to modify to your fitness level and low-impact.

4. Strength Training: You may keep your muscles strong and toned by using resistance bands or small weights. For advice on suitable workouts, make sure to speak with your healthcare provider or fitness professional.

4.3 Recipes that Boost Your Energy

During the second trimester, you might discover that you need an extra energy boost as your baby grows. The following dishes will help you fuel your body:

Black bean and quinoa salad:

Ingredients:

- 1 cup cooked quinoa
- One can have washed and drained black beans
- One cup of fresh or frozen corn kernels
- One sliced red bell pepper
- 1/4 cup finely chopped fresh cilantro
- Lime juice from two
- Add pepper and salt to taste.

Instructions: Mix everything together and squeeze in the lime juice. This salad, which is high in protein, is easy to prepare and gives you a terrific energy boost.

Trail Mix:

Ingredients:

- Cashews, walnuts, and almonds
- Dried fruits, such as cranberries, raisins, and apricots
- Chips made of dark chocolate

Directions: For a quick and energizing snack, combine your preferred nuts and dried fruits.

Green Smoothie:

Components:

- One cup of kale or spinach
- One banana
- Half a cup of yogurt
- One tablespoon of honey
- One cup of almond milk or water

Instructions: Mix every item until its smooth. This nutrient-rich green smoothie will help you maintain a high level of energy.

It can be a great time to try new foods, keep moving, and eat meals that will give you more energy throughout the second trimester. Accept this stage of your pregnancy and relish each wonderful moment. We'll keep giving you wholesome and delectable recipes in the next chapters to help you maintain your health and wellbeing during this incredible journey.

Chapter 5: Power Foods for the Third Trimester

The latter stages of your amazing pregnancy experience begin in the third trimester. It's critical to concentrate on eating meals that are wholesome and can support both your health and your baby's development as they grow quickly and your body gets ready for labor and delivery. This chapter will cover power foods, which can help ease typical pregnancy discomforts, help you get ready for birth, and give you with recipes to sate your cravings.

5.1 Getting Ready for Delivery and Labor

Your body changes significantly as your due date draws near in order to get ready for delivery. An easier labor and delivery procedure can be encouraged and these improvements can be supported with proper diet. Think about including these power items in your diet:

1. **Omega-3 Fatty Acids:** Foods high in omega-3 fatty acids, such walnuts, salmon, and flaxseeds, can help lower inflammation and support a happy pregnancy.

2. **Protein:** The amino acids required for labor muscle

contractions are found in lean protein foods like chicken, turkey, and legumes.

3. Whole Grains: During prolonged labor, whole grains such as quinoa, brown rice, and oats can offer prolonged energy.

4. Fiber: Fruits, vegetables, and whole grains are high in fiber and can help avoid constipation, which is a frequent symptom during the third trimester of pregnancy.

5. Calcium: A sufficient diet of calcium promotes the health of bones and muscles. Dairy products and plant-based milk with added nutrients are great sources.

5.2 Relieving Pregnancy Pain

Some discomforts that are perfectly natural but might be difficult to manage can arise during the third trimester. The following foods may help ease some of the usual discomforts associated with pregnancy:

1. Ginger: Ginger can aid with nausea and digestive problems. It can be found in tea, sweets, and even foods flavored with ginger.

2. Peppermint: Heartburn and indigestion can be relieved with peppermint tea or mints.

3. Foods High in Fiber: Foods high in fiber, such as bran cereal and prunes, can help ease constipation.

4. Leafy Greens: Rich in magnesium, leafy greens can help ease the pain associated with cramping muscles.

5.3 Recipes to Satisfy Cravings

During the third trimester, cravings are typical. While occasionally giving in to these cravings is acceptable, it's important to do so in moderation. Here are some dishes that sate your cravings throughout pregnancy without sacrificing your health:

Chocolate Banana Smoothie:

Components:

- One mature banana
- Two tsp of cocoa powder without sugar added
- 1 cup of Greek yogurt, plain
- One tablespoon of honey

- Half a cup of almond milk

Instructions: Mix all ingredients together to create a rich, creamy dessert.

Toast with avocados:

Components:

- One juicy avocado
- Whole wheat bread
- A dash of red pepper flakes and salt

Instructions: Spread the avocado on whole-grain toast after mashing it. For a savory and creamy treat, put some salt and red pepper flakes on top.

Homemade Trail Mix:

Components:

- Blended nuts
- Chips made of dark chocolate
- Berry dries
- Flakes of coconut

Instructions: Create a personalized trail mix with your preferred ingredients to satisfy your cravings whenever they arise.

Concentrate on the power foods that can sustain you during this special stage of your pregnancy as you approach the third trimester. As the joyous moment of meeting your new baby draws near, these nutrients will help you stay healthy and comfortable with dishes that will satisfy your appetites. We'll be sharing more delectable and nourishing recipes with you in the upcoming chapters to help you maintain your wellbeing during this incredible trip.

Chapter 6: Special Diets and Dietary Restrictions

You should focus particularly on your nutrition during pregnancy, and this is even more crucial if you have particular dietary requirements or restrictions. We'll look at a range of special diets and dietary limitations in this chapter, including gluten-free and allergy-friendly options, recipes that work for gestational diabetes, and vegetarian and vegan options.

6.1 Vegetarian and Vegan Pregnancy

You can still acquire all the nutrients you and your unborn child need while pregnant and follow a vegetarian or vegan diet. Key factors to keep in mind for both are as follows:

1. Protein: You can get the protein you need from plant-based foods including quinoa, tempeh, tofu, and lentils. To guarantee full amino acid profiles, include a range of these sources in your diet.

2. Vitamin B12: Since animal products are the main source of vitamin B12, you may want to take a supplement or eat foods fortified with B12, including cereals or plant-based milk.

3. Iron: It's important to consume plant-based iron sources such lentils, beans, and fortified cereals. Combine them with foods high in vitamin C to enhance the absorption of iron.

4. Calcium: Leafy greens, fortified tofu, and plant-based milk are good sources of calcium.

5. Omega-3 Fatty Acids: To make sure you're receiving enough omega-3s, eat foods like walnuts, flaxseeds, and chia seeds.

6.2 Gluten-Free and Allergen-Friendly Options

Discovering substitutes that offer vital nutrients is crucial if you have to avoid allergens like dairy or nuts, have celiac disease, or are sensitive to gluten. Here are some things to think about:

1. Gluten-Free Grains: Look into gluten-free bread and pasta options, as well as gluten-free grains like quinoa, rice, and oats.

2. Dairy Substitutes: Plant-based milk substitutes, such as almond, soy, or coconut milk, are a good option if you're trying to avoid dairy.

3. Allergen-Free Protein: If you're allergic to nuts, try getting your protein and healthy fats from seeds like pumpkin or sunflower seeds.

4. Reading labels: Make sure items are free of the allergens you need to stay away from by always checking the labels.

6.3 Recipes Suitable for Gestational Diabetes

Pregnancy can cause gestational diabetes, which is a condition that requires regular monitoring of blood sugar levels. These recipes are intended to assist in the management of gestational diabetes:

Stuffed Bell Peppers:

Additives:

- Bell peppers
- Lean ground turkey or a meat alternative made of plants
- Brown rice or quinoa
- A tomato
- Celery
- Onion
- Seasonings such as basil and oregano

Instructions: Stuff bell peppers with a mixture of lean protein, whole grains, and veggies; bake until the filling is soft.

Zucchini Noodles with Pesto:

Ingredients:

- Spiralized zucchini noodles
- Whether homemade or purchased from a store, seek for a version with less sugar.

Instructions: Combine pesto with zucchini noodles to create a tasty and easy low-carb supper.

Quinoa with Greek Salad:

Components:

- Quinoa Tomatoes with Cucumbers
- Onion red
- Feta cheese or a Greek dressing substitute free of dairy

Instructions: For a filling, low-glycemic salad, toss cooked quinoa with fresh vegetables and a light dressing.

It can be difficult to follow particular diets and dietary restrictions when pregnant, but it is totally doable with the correct preparation and decisions. You can have a happy and healthful pregnancy experience by adopting appropriate recipes and paying attention to your unique nutritional requirements. We will continue to offer you scrumptious and nourishing dishes in the upcoming chapters to help you maintain your wellbeing during this amazing period.

Chapter 7: Creating a Pregnancy Meal Plan

It can be challenging to juggle your regular schedule with the nutritional demands of pregnancy. A organized pregnancy food plan is crucial to guarantee you and your baby are getting the nutrition you need. This chapter will cover how to establish a pregnancy meal plan, offer time-saving advice for soon-to-be working mothers, and list the kitchen necessities that will help your pregnancy go more smoothly.

7.1 Making a Meal Plan for Pregnancy

A pregnancy meal plan may guarantee that you're getting a range of nutrients, help you keep organized, and help you choose healthier foods. This is how to make one:

1. Balanced Diet: A balanced diet should consist of a range of foods, such as whole grains, fruits, vegetables, lean meats, dairy products, and dairy substitutes. Plan for multiple small meals and snacks throughout the day to maintain energy levels.

2. Nutrient Prioritization: Prioritize your nutrients by making sure that your meal plan includes foods high in folic acid, iron, calcium, and protein—all of which are vital during pregnancy.

3. Hydration: Make sure you have plenty water to drink during the day. During pregnancy, it's important to stay hydrated.

4. Snack Selection: To satisfy cravings without reaching for processed or sugary foods, make a plan for healthy snack selections.

5. Supplements: If your doctor advises taking prenatal vitamins, make sure to schedule them into your regimen at the right intervals.

7.2 Time-Saving Advice for Expecting Busy Moms

Being pregnant usually means having a hectic schedule, whether you're managing multiple duties, working, or caring for other children. The following time-saving advice will help you stick to your food plan:

1. Batch cooking: When you have the time, make bigger batches of meals and freeze them in portion-sized freezer bags for later use.

2. Meal prep: Set aside some time on the weekend to prepare some or all of the ingredients for the upcoming week's meals. Prepare grains, chop veggies, and portion snacks to speed up the process of assembling meals.

3. Crockpot or Instant Pot: For preoccupied expectant mothers, the Crockpot and Instant Pot are indispensable culinary tools. Toss in your ingredients first thing in the morning, and by dinnertime, you'll have a delicious, wholesome meal ready.

4. Grocery List and Online Shopping: To save time and lower stress, make a shopping list based on your meal plan and place your purchases online.

5. Assign and Accept Assistance: Don't be afraid to approach your spouse, relatives, or friends for assistance. They can help you prepare meals or handle other duties, freeing up more time for self-care.

7.2 Essential Kitchen Items for Expectant Mothers

A well-stocked kitchen can make cooking and food preparation easier, which will ease the transition into motherhood. Here are a few kitchen necessities for new mothers to have:

1. Blender: Smoothies, soups, and purees are wonderful options for meals that are easy to digest and can be made with a high-quality blender.

2. Food processor: When preparing items, a food processor can aid with chopping, slicing, and dicing, saving you time.

3. Steamer: Vegetables can be cooked in a steamer, which keeps their nutrients intact.

4. Slow Cooker or Instant Pot: A slow cooker or instant pot is great kitchen tools for one-pot, hands-free cooking that can save a ton of time.

5. Freezer Bags and Containers: Stock up on freezer-safe bags and containers so you can store cooked meals and cook in bulk.

6. Knife Set: Preparing meals can be done more quickly and safely with a well-made, sharp knife set.

Maintaining your nutritional needs throughout pregnancy can be greatly aided by planning your meals, putting time-saving techniques into practice, and stocking your kitchen with the necessities especially if you have a hectic schedule. You may concentrate on your health and the joy of bringing your new baby into the world by remaining well-organized and prepared. We'll be sharing more delectable and nourishing recipes with you in the next chapters to help you maintain your wellbeing as you embark on this incredible adventure.

Chapter 8: Delicious and Nutrient-Packed Recipes

Making sure you and your unborn child get enough nutrition while enjoying a range of flavors is crucial during your pregnancy. We offer a variety of tasty and nutrient-dense dishes in this chapter to help you maintain your health and wellbeing throughout this incredible adventure. We've got you covered for everything from filling breakfasts to healthy lunches, meals that the whole family will enjoy, and delightful snacks and desserts. We'll also look at some delicious drinks and smoothies to keep you feeling reenergized.

8.1 Mornings with Champions

A hearty breakfast gives you energy and essential nutrients, and it sets the tone for the rest of the day. To get your morning going, consider these options:

1. **Greek Yogurt Concession:** For a filling, high-protein breakfast, top Greek yogurt with granola, honey, and fresh berries.

2. **Avocado and Spinach Scramble:** Diced avocado and baby

spinach combined with scrambled eggs provide a flavorful and nutrient-dense breakfast.

3. Peanut Butter and Banana Smoothie: A creamy, high-protein smoothie can be made by blending ripe bananas, peanut butter, Greek yogurt, and a small amount of honey.

8.3 Lunch Ideas to Get You Through

A midday meal ought to be substantial enough to sustain your energy levels into the afternoon. Consider these lunch ideas:

1. Quinoa and Chickpea Salad: To make a cool, high-protein salad, mix cooked quinoa with chickpeas, cherry tomatoes, cucumber, red onion, and lemon vinaigrette.

2. Veggie Wrap: For a wholesome and filling lunch, wrap hummus, avocado, roasted red pepper, and leafy greens in a whole-grain tortilla.

3. Mango Chicken Salad: For a tropical, high-protein salad, combine grilled chicken, mango pieces, mixed greens, and a zesty vinaigrette.

8.3 Dinners for the Whole Family

The family can get together for dinner and enjoy a filling meal. All of the diners at the table will like these recipes:

1. Baked Salmon with Lemon and Dill: Bake salmon fillets for a tasty, omega-3-rich supper after seasoning with lemon, dill, and a little garlic.

2. Vegetable Stir-Fry: Tofu or lean protein can be stir-fried with a range of vibrant veggies and a tasty sauce to create a filling and nutrient-dense meal.

3. Mediterranean Chickpea Stew: Gently cook chickpeas, tomatoes, spinach, and seasonings to create a flavorful, plant-based stew that is packed with nutrients.

8.4 Snacks and Sweets

It is possible to satiate your urges in a healthy way. Try these treats and nibbles:

1. Homemade Trail Mix: For a personalized trail mix, mix together mixed nuts, dark chocolate chips, dried berries, and coconut flakes.

2. No-Bake Energy Bites: This no-bake, energy-boosting nibbles are made with oats, peanut butter, honey, and micro chocolate chips.

3. Frozen Yogurt and Berry Popsicles: For a cool treat, blend Greek yogurt with fresh berries and a little honey, and then freeze in Popsicle molds.

8.5 Sips and Smoothies

Drink plenty of water and enjoy these tasty drinks and smoothies:

1. Cucumber and Mint Water: For a cool, hydrating drink, add cucumber slices and fresh mint leaves to water.

2. Green Detox Smoothie: For a refreshing green smoothie, blend spinach, banana, pineapple, and a small amount of coconut water.

3. Berry Blast Smoothie: For a tart and sweet smoothie, combine Greek yogurt, mixed berries, and honey.

These recipes are designed to provide flavor and vital nutrients for both you and your infant. These dishes, whether you're having a hearty breakfast, a filling lunch, a delicious supper, a gratifying snack, or a cool drink, are made to promote your health and wellbeing during your pregnancy.

Chapter 9: Postpartum Nutrition

Your diet is still very important as a new mother during the postpartum phase. Your body changed a lot throughout pregnancy and delivery, and your nutritional requirements are still changing. This chapter will address the significance of postpartum nutrition, present suggestions for healing following childbirth, highlight foods that are suitable for nursing, and offer advice on meal planning for the fourth trimester.

9.1 Recovering after Birth

A period of both physical and emotional adjustment follows childbirth. In order to support your body's healing and assist you in adjusting to the new responsibilities of motherhood, proper diet is essential. Here are some crucial things to remember:

1. Hydration: Keep up your water intake to promote healing and to be properly hydrated, particularly if you are nursing a child.

2. Balanced Diet: It's critical to eat a diet full of complex carbohydrates, lean protein, and a range of fruits and vegetables. Your strength will return, your hormone balance will be supported, and your postpartum healing will be aided by these nutrients.

3. Iron and calcium: Depending on your situation, you could still require enough of these elements to make up for any reserves that were lost during pregnancy and childbirth.

4. Self-Care: Taking care of your new born should come first, but don't neglect to take care of yourself. Eat regular, well-balanced meals, and whenever you can, schedule downtime for relaxation and self-care.

9.2 Breastfeeding-Friendly Foods

Your body needs more energy and nutrients to create breast milk, thus your nutritional demands are still higher if you are breastfeeding. Consider some of the following meals if you are nursing:

1. Oats: Oats have a reputation for helping to support the production of milk. Oatmeal can be had during breakfast or used to lactation cookies.

2. Fenugreek: To increase milk production, fenugreek pills or seeds are frequently utilized.

3. Dark, Leafy Greens: You can incorporate foods high in iron and calcium, like as collard greens, spinach, and kale, into your postpartum diet.

4. Lean Proteins: Protein is crucial for your baby's growth and development as well as for your own postpartum recuperation.

5. Hydration: Maintaining adequate hydration is essential for producing milk. Make it a habit to routinely sip herbal teas and water.

9.3 Meal Planning for the Fourth Trimester

In the days following childbirth, meal preparation can literally save your life. You might not have much time or energy to cook when you have a new baby to take care of. Here are some pointers for efficient meal preparation:

1. Plan Ahead: Make meals ahead of time and freeze them for convenient, fast access to a variety of nutrient-dense options.

2. Snacks: To stave off hunger during those hectic times, always have a stock of nutritious snacks close at hand, such as almonds, dried fruit, and precut veggies.

3. Simple Recipes: Put your attention on quick and simple recipes that call for little prep work, like sheet pan dinners, slow cooker meals, and one-pot meals.

4. Accept Help: Whether it's a home-cooked meal or assistance with duties around the house, don't be reluctant to accept offers of aid from family and friends.

5. Self-Care: Make time for relaxation, exercise, and rest as a top priority. A mother who is well-fed and rested is better able to tend to her new born.

The postpartum phase is a period of adjustment, recuperation, and healing. In order to take the best possible care of your new born and for your own health, you must practice self-care and proper nutrition. Remember to put your health first and give yourself enough nourishment as you start this new chapter in your life. We gave you a ton of recipes and advice in the earlier chapters to help you stay healthy during your pregnancy. In order to guarantee that you and your child receive the finest care possible during the postpartum period, keep using these resources to nourish yourself.

Chapter 10: Your Healthy Pregnancy Journey

It's important to take stock of your pregnancy as it draws to a close and be ready for your baby's birth. As you begin this life-changing and exquisite stage, we'll go over the significance of maintaining an active lifestyle during pregnancy, practicing stress management and self-care, and getting ready for motherhood in this last chapter.

10.1 Staying Active during Pregnancy

Your physical and mental health during pregnancy depends on you continuing to stay active. Exercise can assist with weight management, enhancing sleep quality, and easing common pregnant discomforts. Here are a few safe methods to continue exercising while expecting:

1. Prenatal Yoga: Prenatal yoga programs put a strong emphasis on breathing techniques, relaxation, and flexibility, all of which are helpful throughout pregnancy and labor.

2. Swimming: Swimming s a full-body, low-impact exercise that helps relieve the extra weight of pregnancy and is kind to your joints.

3. Walking: Taking a daily walk is a simple yet effective way to stay active. It is adaptable to your fitness level and low-impact.

4. Strength Training: You may keep your muscles strong and toned by using resistance bands or small weights. See your physician or a fitness professional for advice on appropriate workouts.

10.2 Stress Reduction and Self-Care

Being pregnant may be an exciting and demanding time in life. Your wellbeing depends on your ability to control your stress and take care of yourself. Here are some tactics to think about:

1. Meditation and Breathing: Stress reduction and emotional equilibrium can be achieved through relaxation techniques like meditation and deep breathing exercises.

2. Massage and bodywork: Massage therapy, including prenatal massage, can help release tension in the muscles and promote relaxation.

3. Mindfulness: Practicing mindfulness and being in the present moment might help people feel less anxious and more emotionally stable.

4. Support Systems: For emotional support and to discuss experiences and worries rely on friends, family, or support groups.

10.3 Getting Ready to Be a Mom

It's critical to get ready for motherhood as your due date draws near. Your life will change, grow, and face new problems in this new chapter. Here are some actions to think about:

1. Baby Essentials: Make sure you have everything you'll need for your child, including clothes, diapers, a secure cot, and a car seat.

2. Postpartum Support: Take into account your network of postpartum supporters. Who can support you emotionally in the early weeks following delivery, or assist with everyday tasks?

3. Parenting Education: If you're a first-time mother, learning from books on baby care or by enrolling in parenting programs can be quite beneficial.

4. Birth Plan: Let your healthcare professional know about your choices and birth plan. Talk about any worries or inquiries you may have.

5. Time for You: Remind yourself that caring for yourself equates to caring for your child. Establish limits and schedule self-care activities, even if your days are busier after becoming a new mother.

Pregnancy is a journey of change and development for both you and your unborn child. You can guarantee a healthy and happy start to motherhood by maintaining an active lifestyle, controlling your stress, and taking care of yourself. Remain joyful and confident as you embrace the impending changes, and never forget that you are ready to welcome your child into the world. I hope you enjoy this incredible adventure and that becoming a mother brings you endless joy and love.

Conclusion

Celebrating Your Healthy Pregnancy

Thank you for finishing "The Ultimate First-Time Mom's Pregnancy Cookbook: Nutrition Guide Recipes for Healthy Pregnancy." This incredible trip you've taken is evidence of your resilience and commitment to your own and your child's health and wellbeing.

We've covered all the important topics for a healthy pregnancy in this eBook, including the importance of diet, being active, stress management, and getting ready to become a mother. You now know how to promote your well-being during this amazing chapter of your life by learning how to prepare a variety of tasty and nutrient-dense foods for your growing kid and yourself.

Your successful pregnancy is a testament to your fortitude, resiliency, and enduring love for your child. Savor every second of this life-changing event, from the blissful first kicks to the anticipation of the arrival of your child. Long after the baby is born, their wellbeing will be impacted by the decisions you make to put your health and theirs first.

Sources of Additional Assistance

It's crucial to realize that you're never traveling alone as you become a mother. The following resources can offer more help and direction:

1. Healthcare Provider: Keep lines of communication open and schedule routine check-ups with your healthcare provider. They are able to track your development and provide tailored guidance.

2. Parenting Communities: Get in touch with other mothers who have similar experiences, queries, and worries by joining local or online parenting communities.

3. Parenting Books: To learn more about infant care, postpartum recuperation, and parenting techniques, thinks about reading parenting books.

4. Postpartum Support Groups: During the postpartum phase, postpartum support groups can offer emotional support and direction.

5. Friends and Family: Rely on your loved ones for guidance and support while you manage the pleasures and difficulties of being a mother.

You have a wealth of materials at your disposal to help you on your journey, and this eBook is just the start. Recall that each pregnancy and parenthood experience is different, and it's acceptable to ask for help and support when you need it.

As you enter the world of motherhood, remember to treasure the moments, acknowledge your strength, and have faith in your ability to provide a caring and loving environment for your child. This is a voyage of unending joy, love, laughter, and hardships. The basis for a lifetime of happiness with your new family member is a healthy pregnancy.

May this eBook be a helpful resource for you during your pregnancy and a wellspring of inspiration as you make a lifetime of memories with your priceless child. Congratulations on your successful pregnancy and the amazing journey that is ahead of you!

About the Author

Dr. Adam C. stands as a beacon of inspiration in the fields of medicine, nutrition, and self-help, with a remarkable journey that exemplifies the transformative power of healthy living. Armed with a professional master's degree in health nutrition and years of experience, Dr. C. has become a guiding light for individuals seeking to embrace vibrant well-being and lead happier lives.

From an early age, Dr. C. navigated through a myriad of health challenges that ranged from genetic predispositions to the pitfalls of unhealthy eating. His personal struggle ignited a flame of determination within him, one that was fueled by the belief that the human body possesses an incredible ability to heal and rejuvenate through the right nourishment. Through steadfast dedication, Dr. C. managed to conquer his own ailments and emerged as a living testament to the transformative potential of a well-balanced lifestyle.

What sets Dr. Adam C. apart is his rich tapestry of experiences, having been deeply immersed in groundbreaking research in health food and diet-related domains. His quest to uncover the hidden treasures of nutrients within our meals has led to groundbreaking revel actions that empower individuals to extract the maximum benefit from their dietary choices. Dr. C.'s research has not only contributed to the scientific community but has also served as a roadmap for countless individuals striving to optimize their health.

However, it is not just Dr. C.'s academic prowess that has touched lives it is his unparalleled compassion and empathy that truly make him a beacon of hope. His personal journey of triumph over adversity infuses his guidance with an authentic understanding of the challenges his readers and patients face. Dr. C. doesn't just prescribe nutritional plans; he fosters a deep connection with his audience, instilling in them the confidence to embark on their own transformative journeys.

Dr. Adam C.'s holistic approach reaches beyond the confines of traditional medicine. His insights have translated into self-help resources that empower individuals to take charge of their wellness narrative. His words resonate on paper as they do in person, making his books not mere guides, but trusted companions on the path to vitality.

In the realm of health and nutrition, Dr. C. shines as a true luminary. His core strengths lie in his ability to synthesize complex scientific findings into practical, actionable advice that individuals from all walks of life can seamlessly integrate into their routines. Dr. C.'s legacy is not just a collection of breakthroughs; it is a testament to the extraordinary potential that lies within each of us to overcome obstacles and embrace a life brimming with health, happiness, and fulfillment.

As an experienced doctor, passionate nutritionist, and empathetic author, Dr. Adam C. continues to transform lives, showing us that the journey to a healthier, happier existence is within our grasp, waiting to be unlocked through the power of informed choices and unwavering determination.